IN THE
CHILDREN'S EYES

By: Magda L. Grindstaff

Table of Content

Introduction

Each year children are diagnosed with cancer and more children are lost to cancer in the U.S. than any other disease.

Cancer doesn't discriminate, it doesn't matter your religion, your nationality, your socio-economic level, or your race...
Cancer can strike at any time.
Every story, every journey that they are going through is different.

When you hear the word cancer...
You feel lost, in shock, helpless, not knowing what will happen next, if you will survive or not.

No one should go through cancer.

What would you do if you were diagnosed with cancer or your loved ones…?
Sometimes you will never know until you face it.

When you start the journey sometimes you will have ups and downs.
Will you hide from your fears…?
Will you be depressed…?
Sometimes you have to fight with these little demons…
Sometimes you have more questions than answers…
So many things are rushing through your mind…
When you see the children that are fighting cancer, you can see that their faith is strong as well, they make every day the best it can be; they are angels sent by God for a reason.

There are so many stories that can break
your heart…
Some survived others; God has a better
plan for them in heaven.

They teach us a lesson.
They teach us to have faith and to seek
God.
See life in other ways.

Life is precious and sometimes we have to
go through tough trials and to see the
miracles of life and how they unfold
through the children's eyes.

DEDICATION

I would like to dedicate this book to all the children that are going through difficult times.
When cancer knocks in your door, do not lose faith, stay strong.
You are all warriors and angels.
God has better plans for you.
 You are all special.

To the parents that are day in and day out in the hospitals, facing tough trials, remember, you are not alone. Do not lose hope, do not lose your faith, it may not make sense right now, as your life unfolds, God will put people in your life to let you see the unseen.

Life is precious, even though your children are going through a bad day; they make each day better with their smiles and live to their fullest. Their memories are precious; it's a keepsake that will stay forever in your hearts.

ACKNOWLEDGMENT

I would like to thank Talia Castellano, Avalana Ruth, The movie Letters to God and to all the children that they left too soon.
They motivated me to write this book.

I've seen their stories that have touched and changed so many people in so little time.
They are all angels that God sent to us to see the unseen.

The Truth 365 is a documentary film that will educate millions of people to mobilize and to be the voice for all the children facing this reality and the critical need for funding on pediatric cancer research.

They show us the stories of so many children fighting different types of cancer.

I also like to thank my mother in law, Eva Grindstaff, for helping me.

CANCER FACTS

Cancer is the leading cause of death by disease in children and adolescents in the United States. (Source: National Cancer Institute)

Each year in the United States, approximately 13,500 children and adolescents younger than 20 years of age are diagnosed with cancer. (Sources: Center of Disease Control and Children's Oncology Groups)

If you want to know more about the cancer facts please visit the following sites to educate yourself about childhood cancer.

http://www.cancer.org/cancer/cancerinchildren/detailedguide/cancer-in-children-key-statistics

http://www.thetruth365.org/cancer-facts/

http://www.cdc.gov/cancer/dcpc/data/children.htm

http://www.cancer.gov/cancertopics/factsheet/Sites-Types/childhood

POEM
My Angel of Life

MY ANGEL OF LIFE

By: Magda L. Grindstaff

Dear mom,

You are protecting me

with your loving hands.

Your kiss...is warmth

enough to revive my spirit,

to keep fighting.

I hear you plead...

I hear you cry...

When you lift me up and

put me against your chest

I felt your warm body;

I felt and heard your heart
beats.
Mom,
You gave me a CPR of life.
Everything that you are,
you are my angel and I
came back for you.
You guide me through the
light
to come back to you.
I feel safe.

I told God that you are my
protecting and loving angel,
she cares.
God; give me another
chance
A second chance
To live
To love
To laugh
Let me experience
something new.
You never gave up on me.
Thank you mom

For your faith

For your strength

For loving me

You are my Angel of life.

And the story starts...

Mom and dad are waiting for the miracle of life about to happen.
Their lives start to unfold into an excitement; beautiful feelings are rushing through their minds.
They are preparing the room, unknown if it's a boy or a girl, others already know.

For some, their child arrived in 9 months, for others comes earlier.
As mom and dad welcome the most beautiful miracle of life, she covers her baby with the utmost love, tenderness and carefulness, she kisses her newborn child.

The baby started crying, mom started to smile because a new life is about to start.

"A baby is a gift of life that God has given you to protect them, to guide them and whenever they are ready, to let them fly".

As the happiness surrounds the room, the family and friends welcome the child to their home.
What a blessing.

They witnessed and recorded the first walk, the first words; They captured all the great memories of childhood.
They took the child to the first school.
Parents are so excited that their child is doing great.
Then suddenly, something happened; the child has a fever, has an unknown pain, is vomiting and feeling weak.

Mom rushed her child to the hospital, crying, desperate not knowing what is going on.

The doctor came out of the room and tells the mom that they don't know what is causing the illness and the mom asked the doctor to do everything possible, demanding for more analysis necessary to find out about the illness.
The doctor then agrees, the nurse came to the room to take her child to prepare for testing; but before the nurse took the child away, mom kisses her Childs' forehead and prays that everything is OK.

Tears start falling as she watches the nurse take her child away.
As mom awaits, her family comes rushing to find out what was going on, her husband has to leave work to see his child, you can see his face is full of worries, fear, not knowing what is happening.

The doctor came with the news, "Your child has cancer"

The word that no one wants to hear, it is frightening, it is shocking like waves crashing down upon the rocks, it feels like the whole world is falling apart and nothing or no one could make it better, not knowing what is next, what now, what then.

There are more questions than answers and most of the time we lose our way.

Now they have to face tough trials.

Their life has changed forever.

Parents time are torn between hospitals visits, work and home.

Brothers and sisters feel left out, it happens so fast that they don't understand the truth of the matter.

The parents hug…

They cry…

They feel helpless, to see their child getting weaker; their pain is everybody pain.

They cry in silence…

They don't want their child to see they are suffering but is noticeable and somehow the child know.

They are all facing difficult times, looking for words of comfort, to cope with this heavy burden.

Parents are amazed on how their child gets up and keep the smile so vividly, gleaming the room and everywhere they go.

  They know more than we do, is like they have an old soul, and they are here for a purpose.

Sometimes parents cry out a river, with so much pain that

they can't bare; the thought of losing their child, they think to themselves "it is my child" and the constant question rises "WHY?"

God put people in their life to help them face this tough journey that they have to go through day by day.

They met people along the way with the same pain.

They share the different journeys they have been facing.

They learn that they are not alone.

It is difficult to explain the feelings; they are so deep that most of the time they cannot be explained.

In the Children's eyes...

They see how their life changes, missing out on school and friends.

The treatment is taking over their lives.

They will be poked with needles, exposed with harmful chemicals and radiation.

They will lose their hair, eyelashes, eye brows, and lymph's are remove and their organs cut out.

The path to survival it is unknown…

Some will survive but others will not.

But the ones that do survive, they have to face the secondary effect of all the drugs they've being exposed to.

They may develop a secondary cancer, heart disease, infertility and so many others…

Now they have to fight harder than ever before.

In the Children's eyes...

Their tears keep falling, they feel the pain…

The constant battle…

They face the darkness…

It is a heavy burden, what they have to go through and sometimes they feel alone, when mom or dad cannot be with them and they have to be strong on their own.

Sometimes they don't understand what is going on.

Sometimes they have to fight their own thoughts and feelings…

Most of the childhood is gone too fast and they grow up to be an adult in this short time.

The storm keeps pounding so hard, they cry, they feel the pain, their body is so fragile and they feel the lightning strike through their veins, but now they can see through the rain… They are fighting their way… They are trying to hold on… Somehow they find their strength from within, their faith is getting stronger.

And then the Child talks to
Mom:

"Mommy; Why I have so much
pain?
Mommy;
I want to live; I want to be
somebody…"

It is normal to want to live and
they say that everything is
going to be OK at the end.
But everything stops when the
child has cancer.

In the Children's eyes...

They spent most of their childhood in the hospital instead of playing outdoors their favorite sports with friends.

It is hard when you hear the bad news keep coming and sometimes you lose it and sometimes you say things that you didn't mean; you hurt someone with your words.

Sometimes out of desperation, you take it out on someone, looking to blame, since you feel helpless, you feel so tired being in and out of the hospital; see your child to go through, tough days.

In the Children's eyes...
Their pain begins…
The child start talking to God
and to mom and then the child
said,
"Oh God, I am scare.
I have to face the chemo,
I don't know what I will feel…
They said that is harmful for
me, they say that is the
alternative they have.
What else is there God?"

"Mommy,
I'm scared.
I feel the pain when they poke
me with needles."

"Mommy,
I feel something burning inside
of me, I am crying, I am crying.
I am cold; I feel so weak, so
sick that I can barely breathe."

"God,
Help me, lift me up, and just get
me through this night.
Help my mommy that
sometimes she forgets to smile
and to laugh again, worrying
about the IV's, the hospital, and
my sickness…
Help her to find the courage,
help her to find her smile again
and that everything will be OK".

In the Children's eyes...

They have to fight the nightmare each day and each night and face it with faith, with courage.

They feel God next to them, telling them that they are not alone, that they are warriors and they are angels.
Even though they feel weak they keep on smiling, turning the bad days into better days.

The best of all is that they show love wherever they go.

Sometimes we lose our way and they show us our way back with hope, with faith and with a beautiful smile.

In the Children's eyes...

They show love even though there is so much pain.

They are an inspiration.

They show us that there is more in this life to it; they show us to never lose faith.

They are so amazing, they are pure, they want us to see how precious life is and they leave us with an amazing gift; memories…
Lessons…

In the Children's eyes...

 Their time is coming slowly; they are fading away, like clouds in the sky.

They are scare to leave, but as the mother tells her child not to be afraid and is OK to let go.

As hard as it seems to be, you see the ray of the sun into the child face, as the child take one last breath and with a smile, the time has come; the child will go to see and be with God.

POEM
THE CHILDS PRAYERS

THE CHILDS PRAYERS

By Magda L. Grindstaff

"Dear God;

Thank you for everything.
For turning my sorrows
into smiles, test into
testimony, and trials into
triumph.
I've being blessed, for all the
miracles that you've shown
me, along the way of my
fight.

I might be facing a tough day, but as long you are by my side,

 I have nothing to worry, I have nothing to fear and I have faith in you my God, that I will rise again.

If I don't make it, I am sure you have a better plan for me in heaven. Help my family and friends to find the courage to face tomorrow. Amen."

When we are sick or hurting, we often wonder "WHY?"

God can see things that you can't. It may not make sense right now, but one day, when God's whole plan unfolds, you will see what God has for you.

In the Children's eyes...

Their faith and courage inspire others to battle cancer as God's warriors.

As the child reach and gets closer to God, everything turns into a beautiful miracle for some, but for others, God has a better plan in heaven for them.

In the Children's eyes…

They touch our hearts in every way, to teach us, to learn from them, to believe, to have faith.

Even though they were dying, they still manage to live their life to the fullest.

2 Corinthians 3:3 NIV
"You are a letter… written not with pen and ink but with the Spirit of the living God."

In the Children's eyes...

They have seen worst day,
Sometimes they have to fight
with the little demon voices
telling them, to give up…
But their courage roars to keep
fighting that they are stronger,
they are special warriors send
by God with the purpose; to not
give up.

In the Children's eyes…

They teach us to be a better person.

They teach us love.

2 Corinthians 1: 3-4

*"Praise be to the God and Father of our Lord Jesus Christ, the Father of compassion and the God of all comfort, **4** who comforts us in all our troubles, so that we can comfort those in any trouble with the comfort we ourselves have received from God".*

In the Children's eyes…

They learn to fight;

To fight with bravery,

To fight with joy,

With faith,

With hope,

They never forget to smile.

They teach us to live the
moment.
To appreciate what we have.
That no matter how hard the life
can be, to not let it beat you
down, instead to stand up and
fight.

They are amazing…
They are powerful and they are special.

They teach us to believe,
to stand tall even though there
is so much pain or if they feel
tired, they rise again.
You are not dying, you are
starting living.

They teach us to look at the
good in people.

So many children has touched our hearts with their amazing stories, with their smiles, with letters to God, with Makeup , with music and so many other ways that their legacy is still living with us.

They teach us to live the life to the fullest, that life is rich, life has more to it, you just have to open the eyes and see how beautiful it is.
No one is prepared to go through this journey…they have a long road ahead.

THE LOSS OF A CHILD TO CANCER

The loss of a child is difficult. Parents are simply not supposed to outlive their children and no parent is prepared for a child death.

Parents have different reactions and feelings after the death of a child and may grieve the loss in different ways.
So many feelings rushing through their minds, in disbelief of what just happened, they may feel in shock, confuse in constant denial, anger, overwhelming sadness and despair.
Nothing makes sense right now and they search for answers every day.

Feelings of bitterness and unfairness at a life left unfulfilled.
Resentments…

Grieve may come and go like waves; only time will tell.

Now it is your time to help your surviving child during this time of grief, to talk about it, be open even though it is hard.

Join community and other Parents that have being there. They will help you to bring hope in your life.

You should expect that you will never really get over, sometimes the death of the child make you rethink your priorities and reexamine the meaning of life.

In the Children's eyes...

They change your life; they show you new ways to love, new things to find joy in and new ways to look at the world. Their legacy continues on after the death.
The memories of joyful moments you spent and the love you share with your child will live on and always be part of you.

Remember what they teach us, the value of life that the human spirit has the ability to overcome any adversity and to soar to the other side.

Create a legacy in loving memory of your child.

Something to remember each day and what they did that has inspired you to find the meaning of life again.

In the Children's eyes...

They have touched the hearts of strangers, families and friends; who has seen miracles of hope and their inspirations to others that will continue to fight on finding the cure to defeat this monster who is taking the life of so many innocent children.

Poem, Mommy

MOMMY

By: Magda L. Grindstaff

Mommy

I love you

I'm scared...

I know there is something

wrong with me.

I see you plead...

I see you cry...

I see your pain...

An Angel came to me
and told me what was
going on and not to be
afraid.
Mommy,
I feel the pain, when they
poke me with the needles.
I feel something rushing
through my body, is a
burning sensation...
 I am cold...
I feel sick Mommy

Please Mommy;
 make them stop...

The Angel came again,
telling me that he has a
message from God, telling
me to have faith that He
has something better for
me in heaven.
Mommy;
God told me not to be
afraid; I can feel his
presence...

I don't feel any more pain.
Mommy;
God said to have faith and
to believe in Him, to see
how precious life is.
Mommy;
Even though I am no longer
here with you;
I will always live in your
heart.
Cherish every memory I
leave behind and create a
legacy that will inspire and

help others to fight and to
find a cure.
Mommy;
I feel the peace
It's a beautiful feeling...
I thank you mommy for
loving me,
For being there for me,
For being strong in these
tough trials, even though
the fear was trying to
defeat you but your faith
started roaring within you.

Mommy;
I want to tell you
that I am not dying
I am living.
My spirit now soars into
the heavens like eagles.
I ask God for permission to
hug you...
You will feel the breeze
whispering "Mommy I love
you, I will be OK, please
don't cry"

Mommy;

I know to say goodbye to me,

It is the hardest thing to do.

Be strong.

Find the peace Mommy like you always have, celebrate the great things I left behind.

Mommy;

Look at the sky

I will be the brightest star
shinning in the dark.
 I will always be in your
memories and in your
heart.
I love you Mommy,
I will now be in Paradise.
Running free of pain, but I
will be looking down on
you, like an Angel by your
side.

It is now our time to spread the word for more awareness and to find the cure, for all the children.

There are so many Childhood Cancer Organizations that you could help.

Here are a few of them.
Donate to:

Arms Wide Open Childhood Cancer Foundation
http://www.awoccf.org/

Angels for Talia
https://www.facebook.com/angelsfortalia

St Jude
http://www.stjude.org/about

St. Baldrick's
http://www.stbaldricks.org/

The Pediatric cancer research, are in critical need of funding.

Let's make childhood cancer research a
NATIONAL PRIORITY.

ABOUT THE AUTHOR

Born and raised in Puerto Rico.

Orocovis is my hometown, surrounded with beautiful mountains, located in the heart of Puerto Rico.

I use to read poems when I was a kid from famous poets, like Julia de Burgos, Gabriel Garcia Marquez, Alan Poe, Gonzalo Baez and so many more.

Then I start to write, sometimes my subconscious mind delivers all this beautiful feelings, when I hear someone struggles, the loss of someone you love or if I hear a beautiful song that inspire me...

As my life unfolds in a very challenging way, it changes me with a blink on an eye.

I realize that I was prioritizing things that didn't matter; I was forgetting the important things in life.

When I was diagnosed with cancer, I start to see life in a different way that I never saw before.

Writing has help me to cope with my emotions, open new doors to see that no one is perfect and that you are not alone.

You have to take one step at the time in this busy life style.

Everyone has struggles in life and is up to us on how that will be like.

Our mind is so powerful.

You get to choose either feel sorry for yourself or see it as a gift, as a purpose, as a challenge, as an obstacle to overcome.

Don't let anyone tell you otherwise.

I found my passion and that is writing.

I hope this help you, to encourage you in any way.

Make your life the most of it, make it beautiful, and make great memories that will stay with you forever.

Thanks for reading!

Magda L. Grindstaff